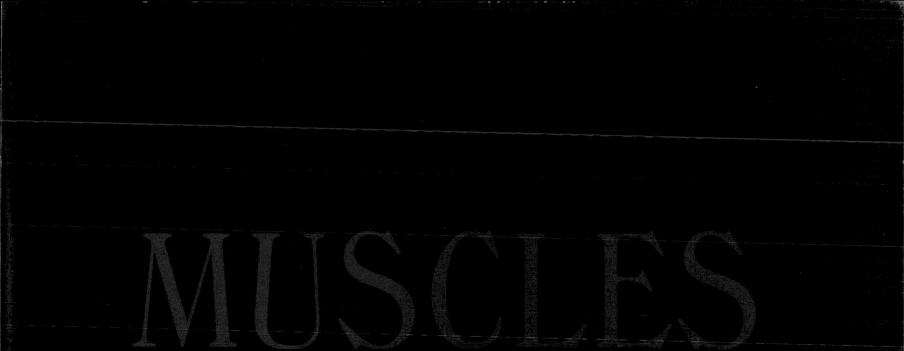

MUSCLES

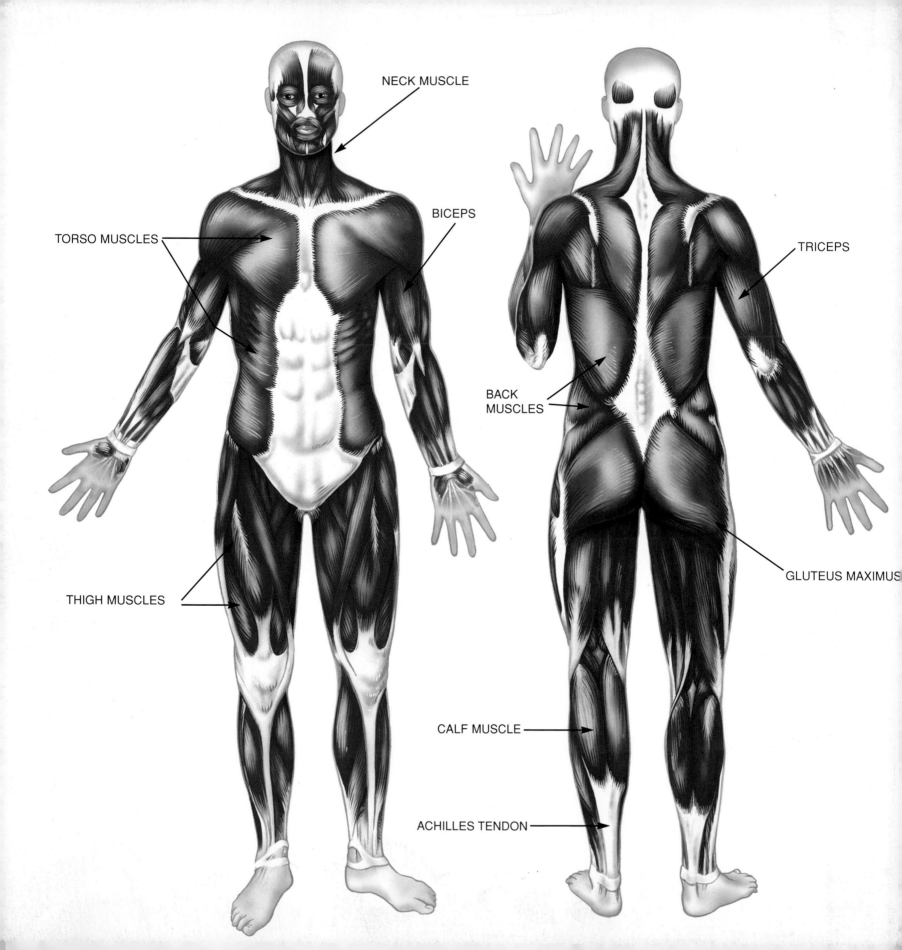

NECK MUSCLE

BICEPS

TORSO MUSCLES

TRICEPS

BACK MUSCLES

THIGH MUSCLES

GLUTEUS MAXIMUS

CALF MUSCLE

ACHILLES TENDON

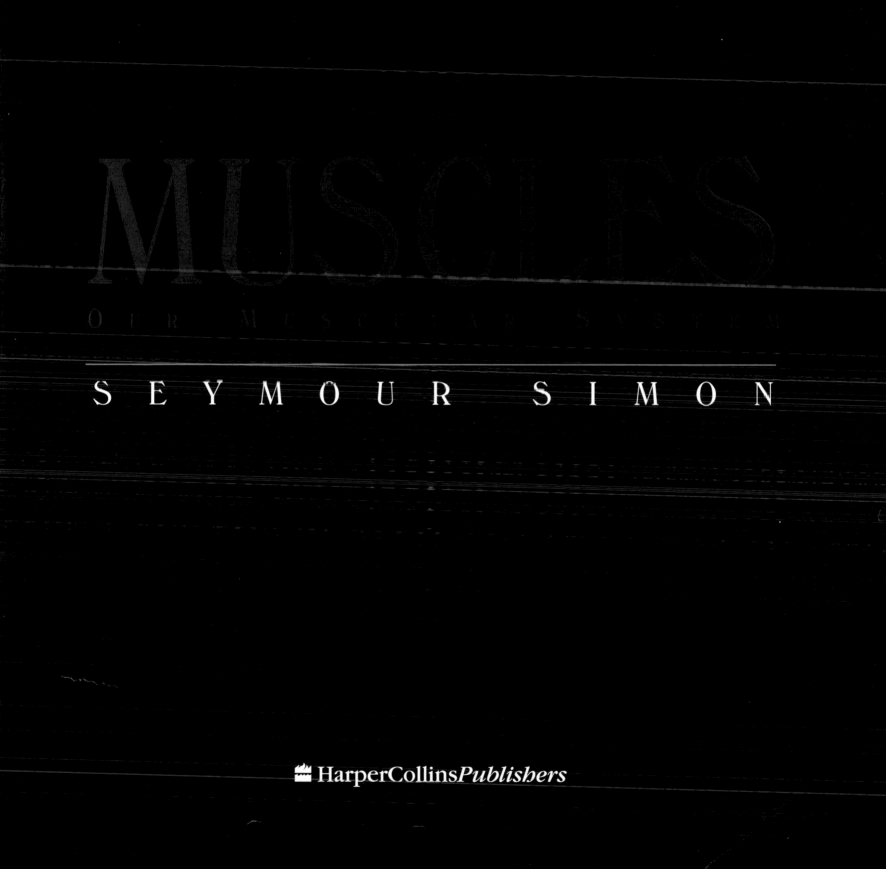

MUSCLES
OUR MUSCULAR SYSTEM

SEYMOUR SIMON

HarperCollins*Publishers*

PHOTOGRAPHY NOTE

Scientists are using fantastic new machines that peer inside the human body to picture the invisible and help doctors save lives. In this book, we see extraordinary views of the interior of the human body. Many of these images were taken by various kinds of scanners, which change X-ray photos into computer code to make clear, colorful graphics. The computer-enhanced pictures of planets beamed back to Earth from distant space use a similar technique. These new ways of seeing help all of us to understand and appreciate that most wonderful machine: the human body.

The author would like to thank Orli R. Etingin, M.D., for her careful
reading of the manuscript of this book.

PHOTO AND ART CREDITS

Permission to use the following photographs is gratefully acknowledged: page 7, John Daugherty/Photo Researchers, Inc.;
page 11, P. Motta/University La Sapienza, Rome/Science Photo Library; pages 12, 15, VU/David M. Phillips; page 13, VU/Triarch;
page 14, VU/Fred Hossler; page 17, Jean-Loup Charmet/Science Photo Library; pages 19, 23, 29, 31, Scott Camazine;
page 20, John Bavosi/Science Photo Library; pages 24, 26–27, 32, Tim Davis/Photo Researchers, Inc.
Art on pages 2 and 8 by Ann Neumann.

Muscles
Copyright © 1998 by Seymour Simon
Manufactured in China. All rights reserved.

Library of Congress Cataloging-in-Publication Data
Simon, Seymour.
    Muscles: our muscular system / Seymour Simon.
        p.   cm.
    Summary: Describes the nature and work of muscles, the different kinds, and the effects of exercise and other activities on them.
    ISBN 0-688-14642-2 (trade) — ISBN 0-688-14643-0 (lib. bdg.) — ISBN 0-688-17720-4 (pbk.)
    1. Muscles—Juvenile literature.   [1. Muscles.   2. Muscular system.]   I. Title.
QP321.S4858   1998   97-44758
612.7'4—dc21   CIP
                                                                                                                                          AC

❖
Visit us on the World Wide Web! www.harperchildrens.com

To the editors and designers
at Morrow Junior Books,
who helped create this series

henever you walk or run, play an instrument, or turn a page of a book, muscles move your body. Even when you're still, muscles are at work, moving your eyelids each time you blink and moving your chest in and out each time you breathe. Your muscles are always moving, even when you are fast asleep.

Muscles make up about 40 percent of a normal person's body weight. Fat, by contrast, makes up only about 10 percent. In addition to the 640 muscles that you control, such as your arm and leg muscles, there are many muscles that you *don't* control. Among these are your stomach muscles, which aid the digestion of your food, and your heart muscles, which keep blood pumping through your body.

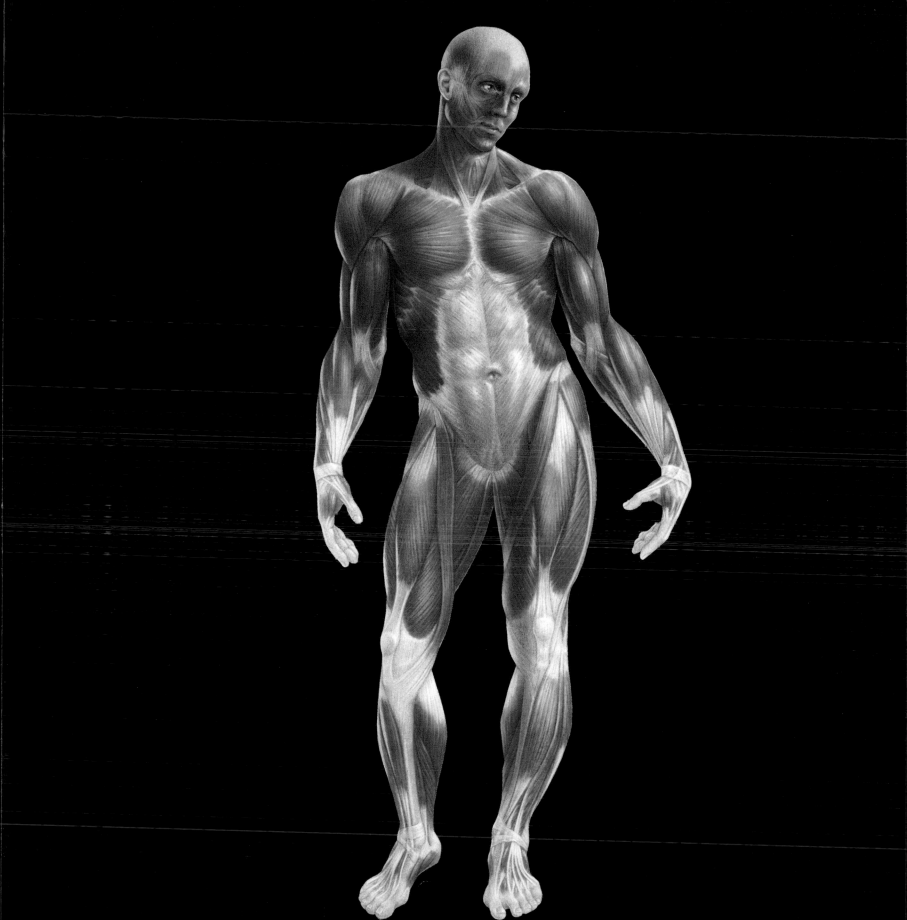

ARM STRAIGHT

ARM BENT

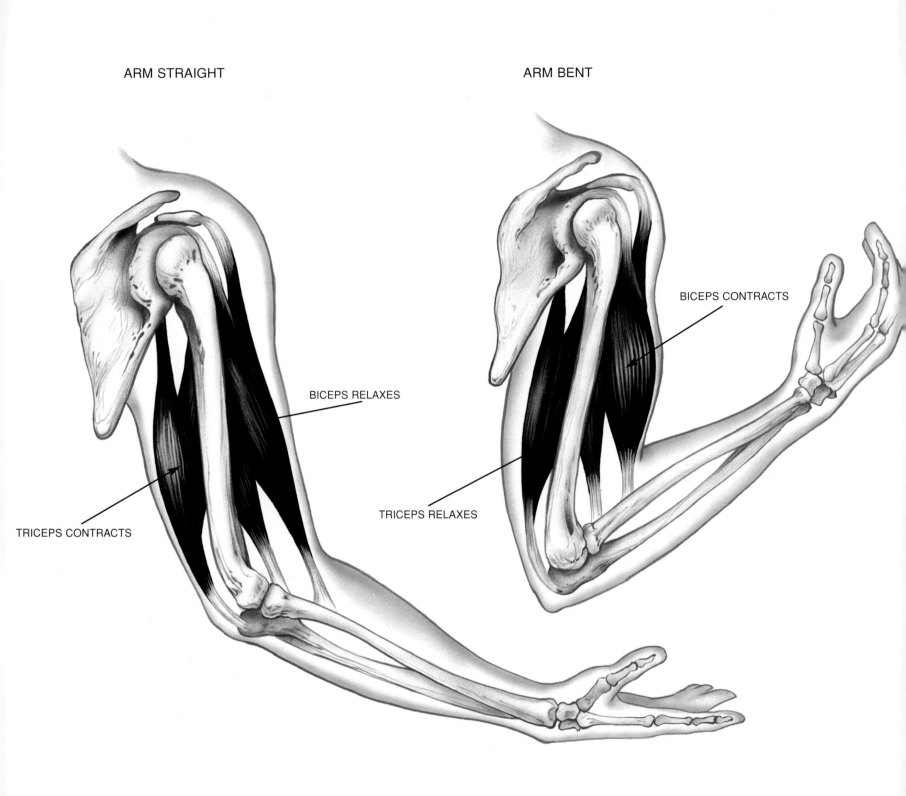

BICEPS CONTRACTS

BICEPS RELAXES

TRICEPS RELAXES

TRICEPS CONTRACTS

Muscles move your body by contracting. When a muscle contracts, it shortens, and that moves the bones to which it is attached. When a muscle relaxes, it lengthens or stretches. Muscles are usually arranged in pairs, so that while one muscle pulls the bone, another muscle relaxes. For instance, when you make a fist and bend your arm, your biceps muscle bends your elbow and your triceps muscle relaxes. Straightening out your arm again causes your triceps muscle to contract and your biceps muscle to relax.

Muscles are attached to bones by narrow, ropelike tissues called tendons. These tendons help to move the bone each time a muscle contracts. Flex your arm back and forth; you can feel the tendons and see them under your skin, moving like tight cords. You can easily see other muscle tendons along the sides of your neck and ankles and behind your knees.

Muscles are made up of bundles of long, thin cells called muscle fibers. A single muscle fiber is thinner than the finest human hair and can be up to a foot long in a large muscle. Despite its size, a muscle fiber is a single cell. Each muscle fiber is made up of thousands of even thinner threads called fibrils, and each fibril is made up of strands of two kinds of proteins, actin and myosin. Proteins are important chemicals that the body uses to make muscles, bones, skin, and other body parts.

Muscles are controlled by electrical signals that come into the muscles from nerves in the brain and spinal cord. When the muscle fibrils receive signals, the actin strands slide past the myosin strands, overlapping the way the teeth of two combs would if you put them together. This sliding action makes the muscle get shorter and thicker, and that moves the part of the body to which it is attached. When the actin strands slide in the other direction, the muscle gets longer and thinner, and it relaxes.

A blood vessel (blue) snakes along muscle fibers (pink).

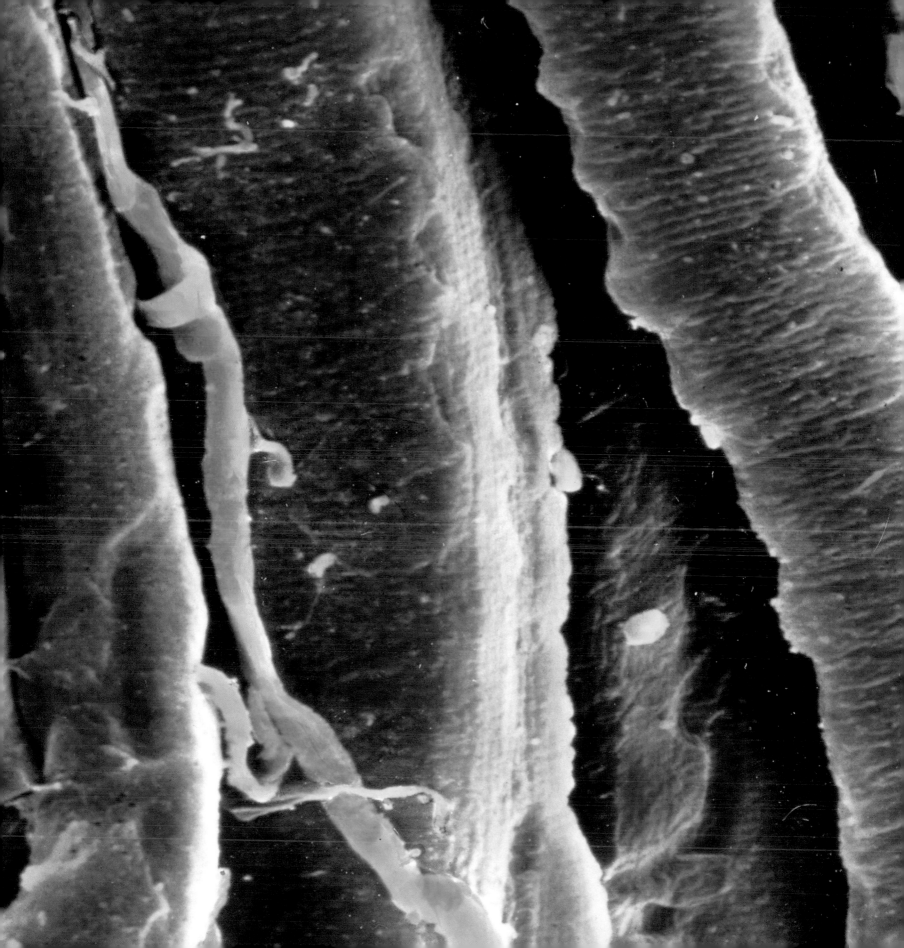

There are three kinds of muscles in the body. Muscles attached to bones are called skeletal muscles. Because you can control your skeletal muscles, they are also called voluntary muscles. These muscles look striped, or striated, under a microscope because the muscle fibers lie next to one another.

Another kind of muscle is called smooth muscle. It is also known as involuntary muscle, because you cannot consciously move it. Unlike skeletal muscles,

These images of skeletal muscle (left) and smooth muscle (right) have been magnified hundreds of times.

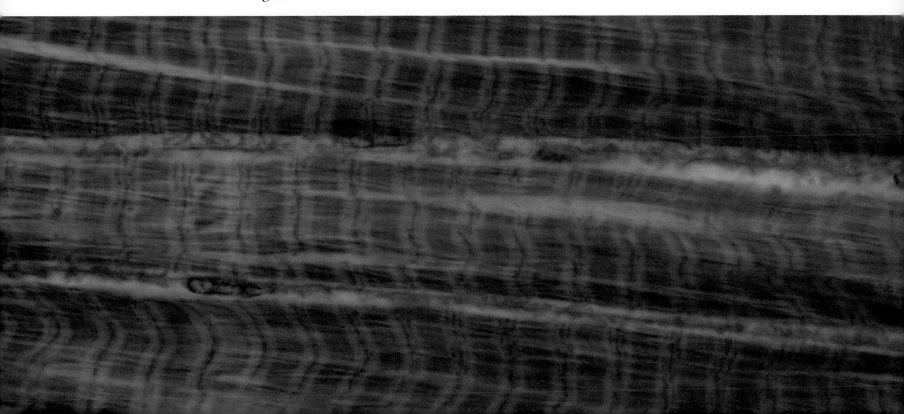

smooth muscles do not look striped under a microscope.

Smooth muscles line the walls of the stomach and the intestines and other hollow tubes, such as blood vessels. These muscles contract the way skeletal muscles do, only much more slowly, and they use less energy than skeletal muscles. As the muscles around the stomach and the intestines contract, they move food through the digestive system.

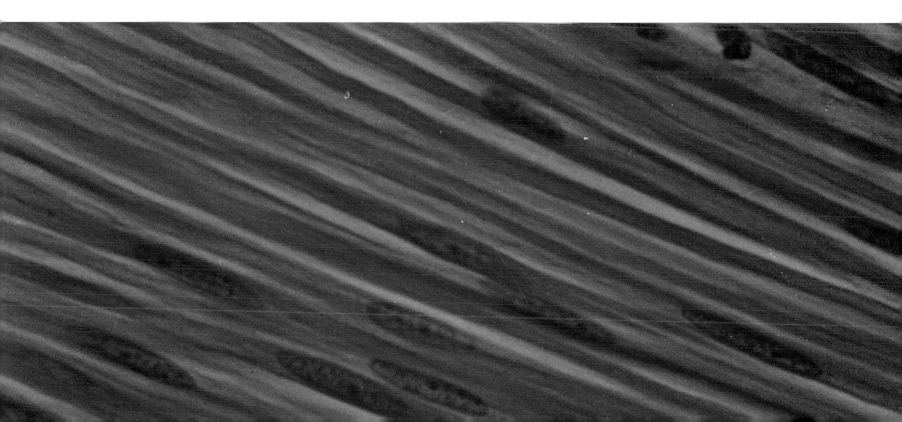

The heart is made of still another kind of muscle. This thick, powerful muscle is called heart, or cardiac, muscle. Cardiac muscle continually contracts and relaxes, pumping blood around your body sixty to seventy times a minute, one hundred thousand times a day. Cardiac muscle never tires, the way skeletal muscles do.

Like smooth muscle, cardiac muscle is involuntary; you cannot consciously make your heart muscles contract. Cardiac muscle has its own built-in rhythm of contracting and relaxing, but signals sent by the brain and nerves can change the rhythm, as can body chemicals called hormones.

Cardiac muscle (below and right) looks striped under a microscope, something like skeletal muscle.

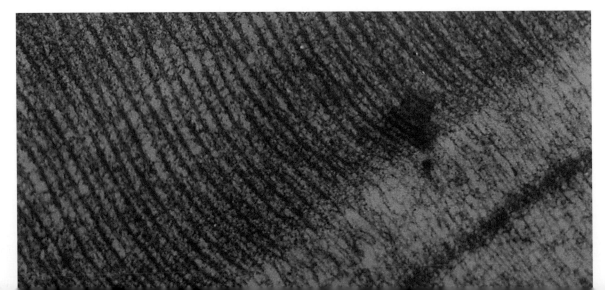

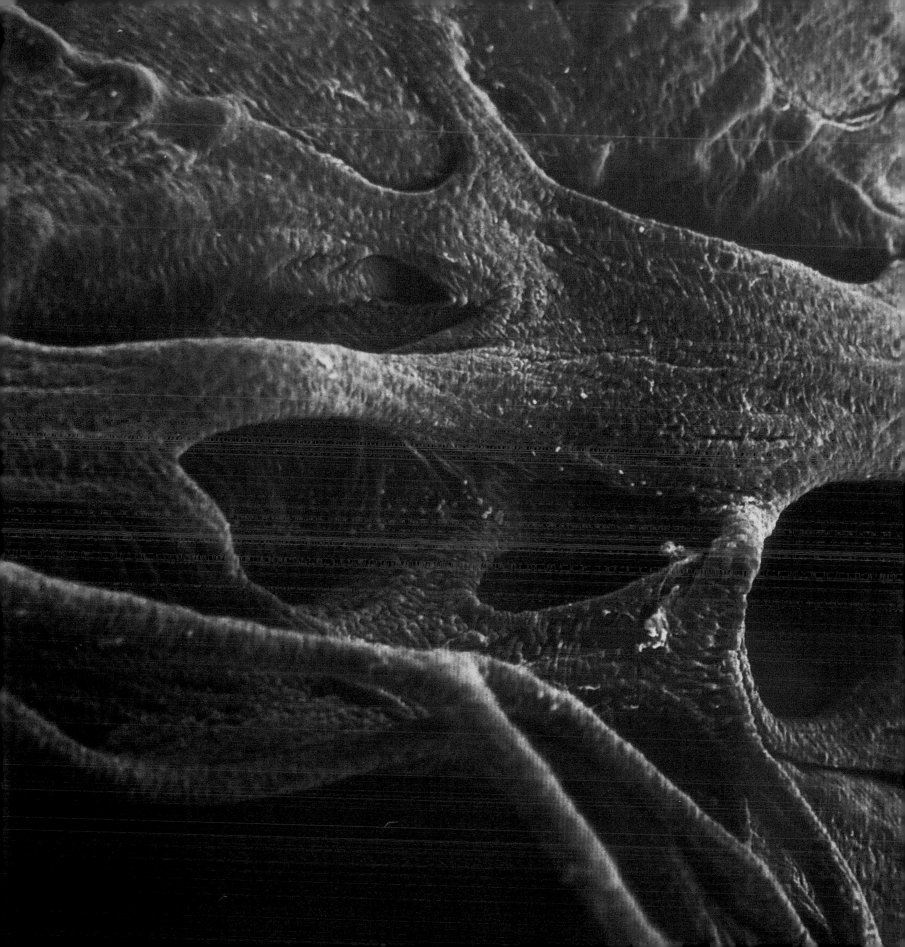

Your face and neck have more than thirty different sets of muscles. Most of them are small and are attached to each other or to the skin, rather than to bones. You use certain muscles to express your moods: When two muscles pull up the corners of your mouth, you smile; if other muscles raise your eyebrows, you look surprised.

Powerful muscles in your cheeks and at the side of your head move your jaw when you speak or eat. Another group of muscles moves the lips in many different directions. The muscles of the lips, together with the tongue and the vocal cords in your throat, produce the many movements and sounds needed for speech.

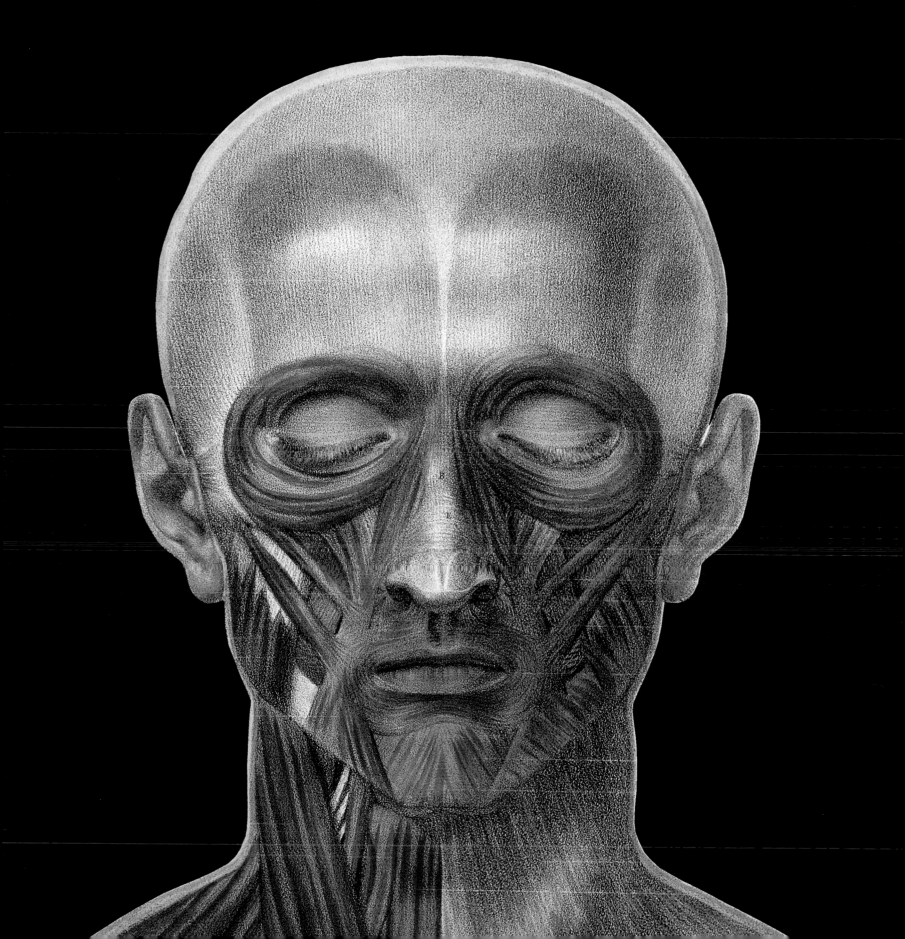

Layers of different muscles surround the central part of your body, which is called the trunk or the torso. The torso contains the heart and lungs and other important organs. Dozens of torso muscles help you to move and breathe and allow you to twist and turn.

Powerful pairs of muscles in your back are an important part of your torso. These help you to stay upright. Other muscle pairs in the front of your torso move your arms and shoulders.

A strong muscle called the diaphragm stretches across your torso from the backbone to the ribs. The diaphragm moves up and down as you breathe in and out. At the same time, muscles between your ribs and diaphragm move your ribs outward and inward as air pushes into and out of your lungs.

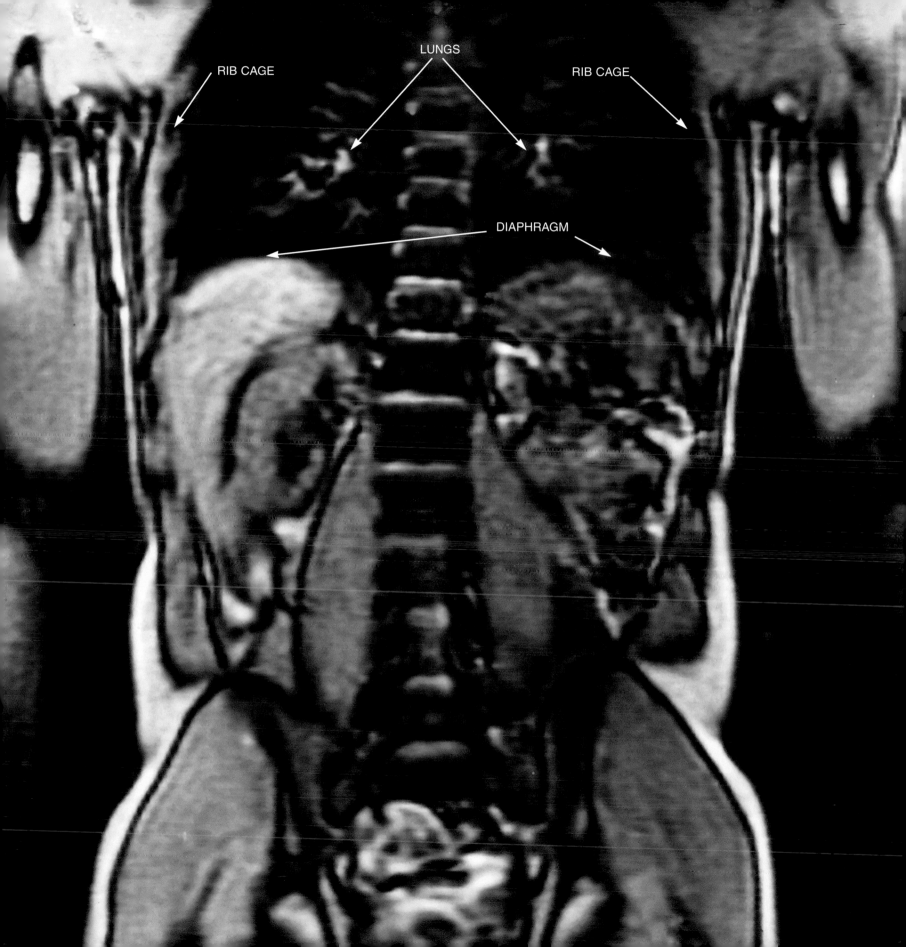

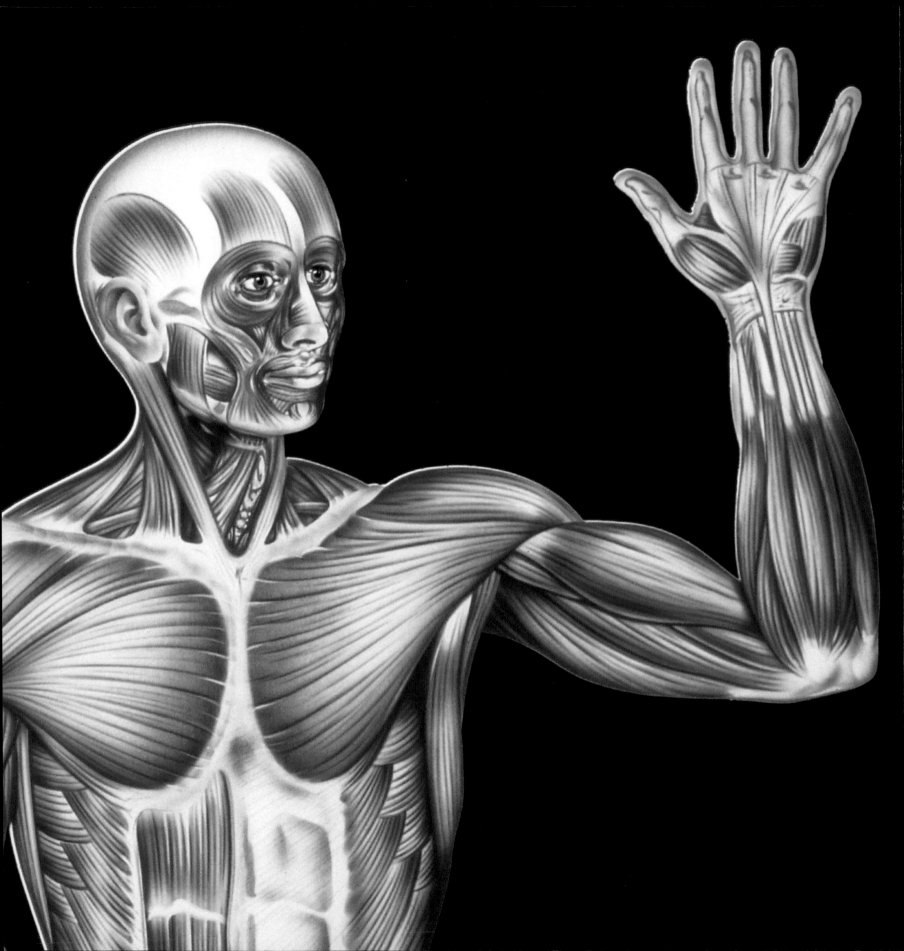

The muscles of your hands and arms work together like a set of delicate tools at the end of a powerful machine. Together, these muscles can gently pick up a tiny feather, or they can support your weight when you do a handstand.

The biceps and triceps bend or straighten the arm and turn it around. When you flex your arm to "make a muscle," the biceps bulge out. There are nineteen muscles in your lower arm and twenty muscles in your hand that control your fingers and your wrist.

The thumb is the most movable part of the hand. Four muscles in your forearm and four in your hand control your thumb and allow you to hold things easily.

The largest and strongest skeletal muscles in your body are in your legs. They help you walk and run, squat down or stand on tiptoes, and they keep you steady when you stand still.

The strong calf muscle at the back of the lower leg makes the foot bend forward and also helps to bend the knee. It is connected to the heel bone by the Achilles tendon, the strongest tendon in the body. The muscles in your feet and toes are like those in your hands and fingers, but the foot muscles are stronger and less flexible.

The biggest muscle in the body, the gluteus maximus in the buttocks, helps to flex the thighs. Other strong muscle pairs in your thighs provide the power to straighten your knees and to swivel your hips each time you stand, walk, run, leap, climb stairs, or sit down.

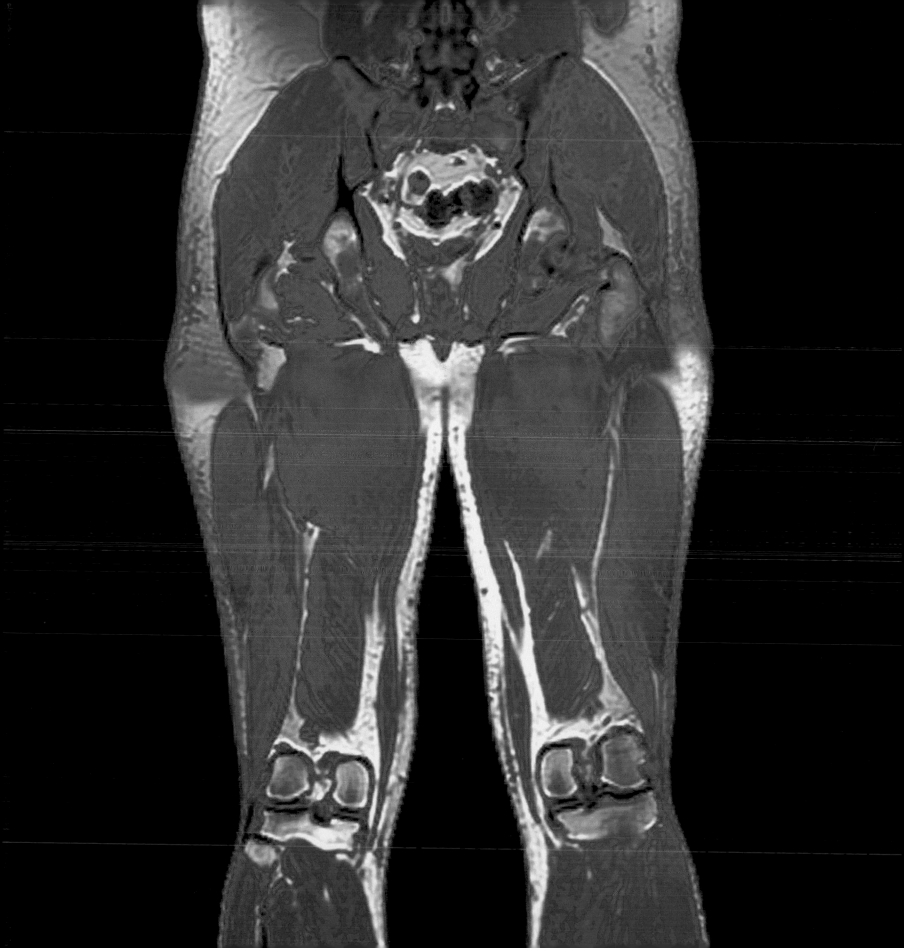

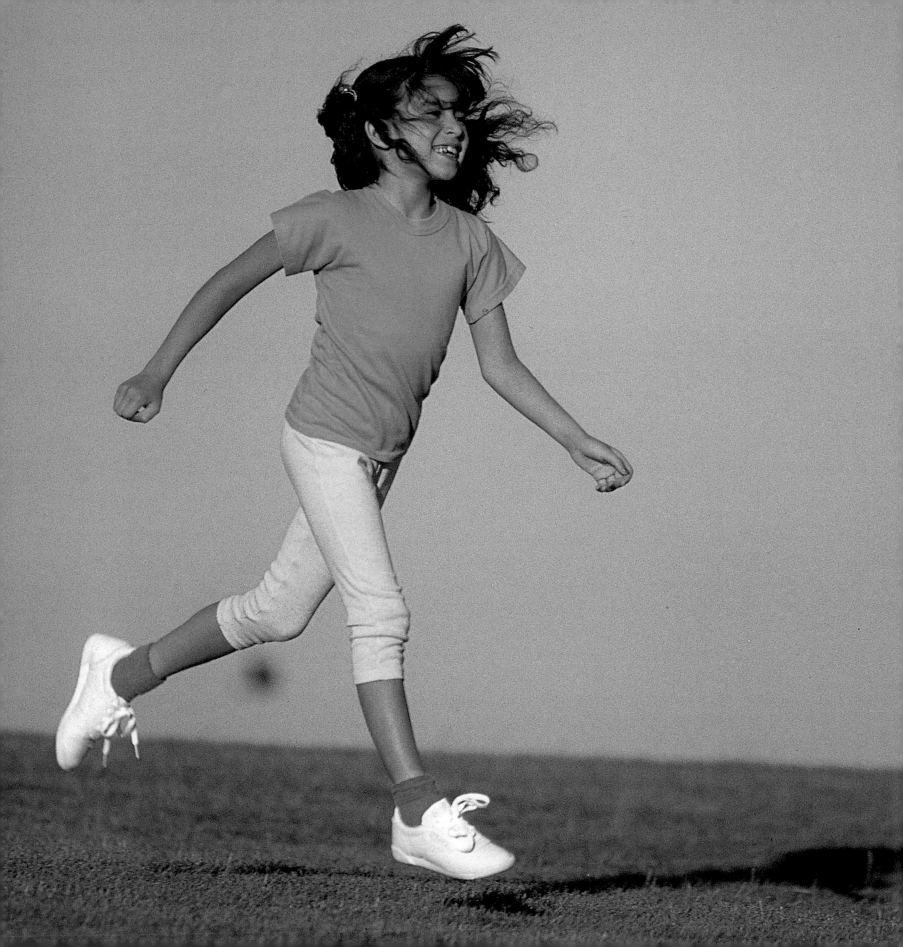

Muscles need food and oxygen in order to work properly. The chemicals in foods build muscle cells and help to repair them if they are damaged. Oxygen, which is carried by red blood cells, enters your muscles and allows you to exercise for long periods of time. The harder your muscles work, the more oxygen they need.

The more a muscle is exercised, the larger the muscle cells become. The blood vessels that enter the muscle widen so that more needed food and oxygen can be supplied. You can use well-exercised muscles for a longer time without tiring them.

Exercise doesn't give you more muscles, but it strengthens the muscles you have and helps keep them working well. Without exercise, muscles shrink and tire easily. This can happen if you are ill and unable to exercise for a long time.

Most athletes like to stretch or warm up their muscles before they compete in a sporting event. Muscles use oxygen and release energy when they are used. This is why you feel hot when you exercise. A warm muscle contracts more quickly and easily, receives more oxygen, and can perform for a longer time than a cold one. Stretching or warming up a muscle can help to prevent injury.

Depending upon the sport, different muscles are used in a warm-up. Runners may stretch out their calf muscles and do some light jogging with brief bursts of speed, while tennis players may stretch their back and arm muscles by hitting a ball easily and without too much power.

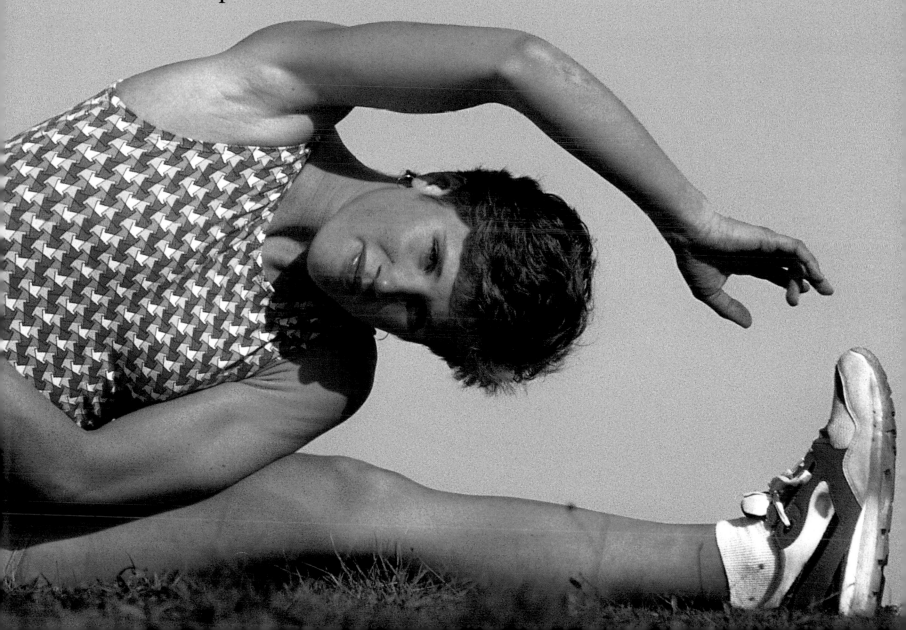

Exercise makes all muscles tired, even strong ones. Clench your fingers and open them again. If you continue to do this rapidly for several minutes, you will eventually have to stop as your muscles tire. That's because your arm and hand muscles are using up oxygen faster than your body can supply it. When this happens, a waste product called lactic acid builds up in the muscle, causing it to tighten or cramp. This can be very painful. The lactic acid usually breaks down in minutes as the muscle rests.

Sometimes muscles begin to hurt because they are strained. A strain usually results from too much use of a muscle, which can tear muscle fibers and cause pain.

Lifting too heavy an object can cause a sudden painful strain in lower back muscles. Cold ice packs on the strain can numb the pain that often follows. A strain is not the same as a sprain, which happens when you injure a joint, such as your ankle or elbow.

This MRI scan shows muscles (pink and red) around the stomach and lower chest. The kidneys (purple) are to the top left and right.

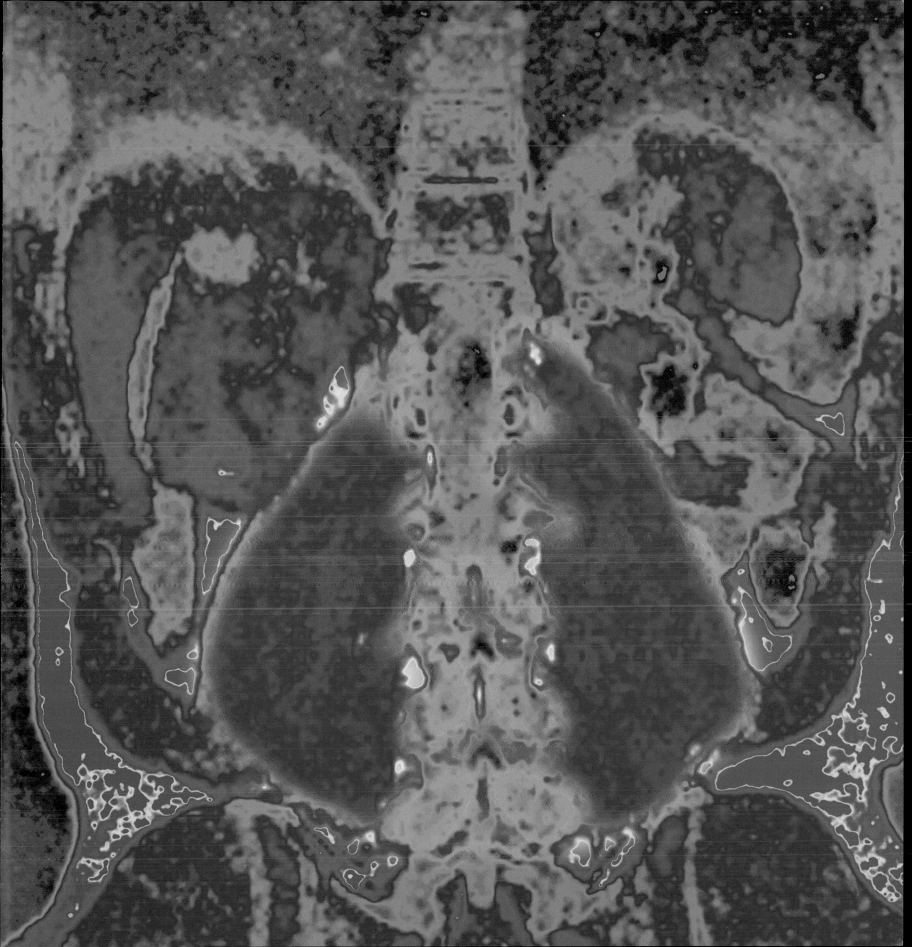

When a muscle is injured, doctors can often look at it without having to perform surgery. New ways of viewing the muscles and the bones help doctors understand what's going on inside the body. Computerized axial tomography (CAT) scans process dozens of X-ray pictures with computers to produce three-dimensional images of muscles and bones. Magnetic resonance imaging, or MRI, scans use powerful magnetic fields that are deflected by tissues that contain a lot of water. Bones don't contain much water, so they do not appear in an MRI, but the surrounding muscles appear very clearly in color images produced by computers.

Other imaging techniques, called SPECT and PET, use radioactive chemicals to show whether muscle tissues are getting enough blood. A test called an EMG measures electrical output and is used to test nerve damage in a muscle.

CAT scan of head

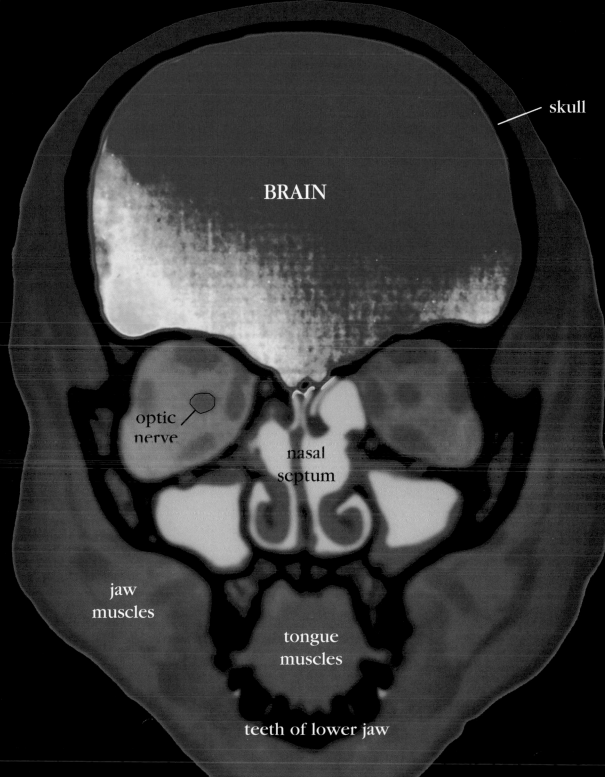

skull

BRAIN

optic nerve

nasal septum

jaw muscles

tongue muscles

teeth of lower jaw

Your muscles adjust themselves to your own movements and activities. There are muscles that you control, and muscles, like those in your heart, that work without your even knowing it. Muscles and bones work together every minute of the day, year after year, to keep your body moving and alive.